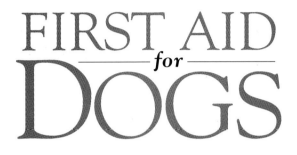

FIRST AID
—*for*—
DOGS

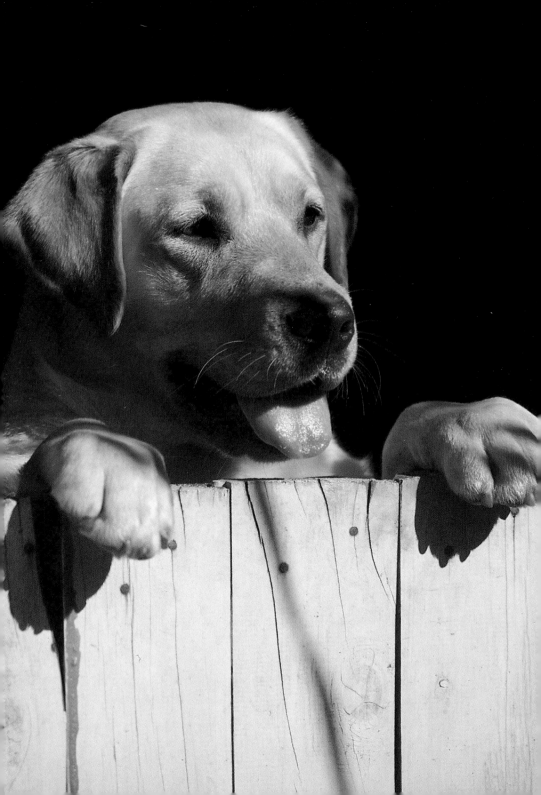

FIRST AID
for
DOGS

The essential quick-reference guide

TIM HAWCROFT
BVSc *(Hons)*, MACVSc, MRCVS

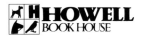
BOOK HOUSE
New York
MAXWELL MACMILLAN CANADA
Toronto
MAXWELL MACMILLAN INTERNATIONAL
New York   Oxford   Singapore   Sydney

Howell Book House
Macmillan Publishing USA
1633 Broadway
New York, NY 10019

Maxwell Macmillan Canada,
Inc.1200 Eglinton Avenue EastSuite 200
Don Mills, Ontario M3C 3NI

Printed in Singapore by Tien Wah Press

Library of Congress Cataloguing-in-Publication Data:

Hawcroft, Tim 1946-
First Aid for Dogs: the essential quick-reference guide/by Tim Hawcroft.
p. cm.
Includes index.
ISBN 0-87605-546-3
1. Dogs - Wounded and injuries–Treatment–Handbooks, manuals, etc.
2. Dogs–Diseases–Treatment–Handbooks, manuals, etc.
3. First aid for animals–Handbooks, manuals, etc. 1. Title
SF991.H29 1994   93-38168 CIP
636.7'08960252—dc20

Macmillan books are available at special discounts for bulk purchases for sales
promotions, premiums, fund-raising, or educational use. For details contact:

Special Sales Director
Macmillan Publishing Company
866 Third Avenue
New York, NY 10022

Macmillan Publishing Company is part of the
Maxwell Communication Group of Companies.

10 9 8 7 6 5 4 3 2 1

CONTENTS

ACKNOWLEDGMENTS

I would like to thank my wife Jan and children Melanie,
Samantha, Damien and Edwina for their support.
My sincere thanks to my father Eric for his diligent assistance in
planning, researching and proofreading, and also to my sister
Judy Shields for transferring my notes to print.
I would also like to thank my partner Dr David Lonergan and
the staff of Gordon Veterinary Hospital — Dr Andrew Morgan,
Dr Sue McMillan and the nurses, Jenifer Reber, Kim Tupper
and Diane Spalding.

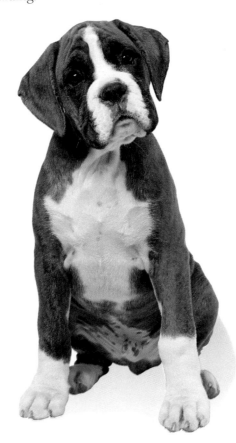

INTRODUCTION

This book of practical First Aid is designed for those owners and dog lovers, in fact for all caring persons, who want to know how to help a dog that is injured or sick, or who want to update and extend their knowledge of First Aid for dogs. The know-how in this book, combined with experience, will give the reader confidence and skill to administer First Aid to a dog in most situations where there is a need for it.

You never know how, when or where you may be confronted with a dog needing treatment for some life-threatening, serious, or simple type of injury or illness. You may already have come face to face with such a situation but been unable to help because of lack of First Aid know-how.

Road accidents, fights, hunting, free running and the home are the most common situations where injuries and illness occur, ranging from fractures, abrasions, near drownings, cuts, bruises, diarrhea, bee stings and grass seed problems to collapse, hypothermia and severe bleeding. Usually, the injury or illness requires some form of First Aid. The increasing frequency and proliferation of such injuries and illnesses in our community underlines a basic need for knowledge, skill and confidence to administer First Aid to dogs as well as to other animals.

To save a life, arrest a worsening condition or just to give some comfort and compassion to a dog in distress, are rewarding experiences.

THE CONCEPT OF FIRST AID

When a dog is hurt or sick, many people do not know how to help. It may be because they do not know how to approach and handle a dog or they do not know how to administer First Aid.

First Aid is not a new concept. Dog owners and others have been practising it for generations. First Aid information has been passed around mainly by word of mouth, but in recent times the media, authors, veterinarians and dog clubs have been disseminating it. The most practical understanding of the term is in its literal interpretation: it is the *First* Aid, help or treatment that is given to an injured or sick dog.

Minor, uncomplicated problems such as a bee sting, grass seed penetration or simple cuts and abrasions may only need a single treatment or, at the most, repetitions of it. The treatment starts and finishes on-site or at home.

Serious and life-threatening injuries and sickness, such as fractures, arterial bleeding and poisoning, need not only immediate First Aid but require further treatment by a veterinarian.

When an injury or sickness occurs at home or, for example, on a roadway, there is usually no veterinarian present. Whatever First Aid is given depends on the knowledge, skill, initiative and confidence of the owner or onlooker and the nature of the dog's injury or sickness. First Aid may range from something very simple, such as comforting the dog, to assessing its condition, perhaps moving it to safety, and then giving it the treatment thought necessary at the time.

Remember that *First* Aid is the first treatment and whatever treatment you can give is better than none at all.

HOW TO USE THIS BOOK

Familiarise yourself with the book's design, the location of various sections and their content. In doing so, you will be able to refer to the book for information in a calm, confident and speedy manner, especially in emergency situations. For ease of reference, we have set out the techniques, injuries and illnesses in alphabetical order. A detailed index in the back of the book will quickly guide you to the information you need.

Of course, the information you require will depend on the situation and your knowledge. You will have to use your own judgement to determine your course of action.

If you are in a situation where a dog requires First Aid and you are unsure of the action you should take, we suggest you consult the following sections in this order:
1. First Aid Priorities (see page 13)
2. The Injured Dog (see page 14)
3. When to Call Your Veterinarian (see page 20)
4. First Aid for Injuries and Illness (see page 50)

These sections offer practical guidance and back-up information so that you can determine what procedure to adopt to treat a particular injury or illness.

Although this book will serve you well in an emergency situation, it is best to be prepared. The purpose of the First Aid Kit section is to prompt you to set up a First Aid kit of your own. Likewise the section on Accident Prevention is there to remind you of the old adage: prevention is better than cure.

To achieve competence in any activity involving skill you must practise. The sections dealing with the Injured Dog and Techniques You Should Know contain procedures you should learn. The more you practise and the closer that practice is to reality, the more proficient and confident you will be when facing a real life situation.

IMPORTANT
Always keep your veterinarian's telephone number handy.

ACCIDENT PREVENTION

ROAD ACCIDENTS
• Always keep your dog on a lead when walking in a traffic area.
• Never let your dog run freely outside the home. Ensure that fences, gates and kennel run are secure.
• Only allow your dog to run freely in open space where there is no traffic danger and the dog is under your control.
• When driving, be prepared for the unexpected if you see a dog by the roadside.

CAR TRAVEL
• If your dog is well behaved, allow it to sit on the back seat. If it is excitable, use either a safety belt specially designed for dogs, a short lead or a carry basket. Do not drive with your dog on the front seat. For some unforeseen reason, the dog may suddenly jump onto your lap or paw at your arm and cause an accident.
• If going on a long journey, stop now and then to allow your dog to relieve itself and to take a little exercise. Take some water with you to give the dog a drink.
• Never leave your dog in the car on a hot summer's day. If you must leave your dog in the car for a short period, ensure that the vehicle is parked in a cool spot and the windows are down slightly to allow some airflow.

ELECTRICAL APPLIANCES
• Take care with electrical cords. Puppies and young dogs like playing with moving objects. For instance, an electrical cord attached to an iron or lawn mower, dangling or wriggling along the ground, is attractive enough for the puppy or young dog to bite in play. Should the dog's teeth penetrate the plastic covering, electric shock results.
• If you plan to use a blow-drier to dry your dog after shampooing, ensure that the drier does not accidentally

fall in the water. Do not rest the blow-drier on the side of the tub whilst the dog is standing in the water.

• A dog, inside the home, may become excited by an animal or person outside and unwittingly charge through a glass door or window. Ensure this cannot happen by giving obedience training in the home, by making the dog familiar with the glass windows or doors which, if possible, should be suitably marked with adhesive tape.

GLASS DOORS AND WINDOWS

• Dogs are natural foragers. Do not leave contaminated food, garden pest pellets and sprays, weed killers and the like exposed and accessible to a hungry or thirsty dog, whether your own or your neighbour's.

POISONS

• Dogs love the freedom to run and play in an open space. Give your dog the opportunity to do so but only under your supervision and control. *If your dog has not been fully obedience trained and is not completely under your control, only allow it to run freely in an area that is fenced and within the law.*
• Never let your dog roam. The free roaming dog is subject to road accidents, poisoning, fight wounds and serious illnesses.
• In some areas there are leash laws. Do not allow your dog to run loose in these areas.

RUNNING FREELY OR ROAMING

• Always walk your dog on a leash. An obedience trained dog will be more responsive and under your control. A dog not on a leash nor fully under control may become excited when seeing another dog or picking up a particular scent and dart off across the street without thought to passing traffic.

STREET SAFETY

• Dogs like water. If you have a swimmping pool, avoid the danger of your dog falling or jumping into your pool and not knowing how to get out. Ensure your dog has sufficient practice in getting out of the pool and knows what to do in the water when no one is around to help.

SWIMMING POOLS

FIRST AID KIT

•Store the First Aid kit in a suitable container, readily accessible, portable, and marked for easy identification.

•Clean any soiled instruments after use and if necessary restock the kit.

•Every six months check to see that all is in working order, for example, test the torch (flashlight) batteries.

•The kit should contain:

- Antibiotic powder

- Antiseptic wash

- Eye dropper

- Gauze swabs

- Hydrogen peroxide 3%

- Mercurochrome (antiseptic solution)

- Paraffin oil

- Roll of cottonwool (absorbent cotton)

- Roll of adhesive bandage (2.5cm (1in) or 7.5cm (3in) wide)

- Roll of gauze bandage (2.5cm (1in) wide)

- Scissors (sharp, pointed, 10cm (4in) long)

- Syringe (plastic, 20mls)

- Thermometer (same as type used for checking human temperature)

- Tincture of iodine (anti-bacterial, anti-fungal solution)

- Torch (flashlight)

- Tweezers (forceps)

- Vetwrap

FIRST AID PRIORITIES

- Keep calm and work methodically.
- In any severe or critical injury or illness, treat shock by keeping the dog calm and warm (see page 89).

1. Life-threatening injuries or illness

- First treat life-threatening conditions. Such signs as:
- Severe bleeding (blood pulsating or flowing freely from a wound) (see page 61).
- No sign of breathing (see page 45).
- No heartbeat (pulse) (see page 33 and 45).

2. Non-life-threatening injuries or illness accompanied by severe pain

- Next treat injuries or illness, such as a fracture or extensive burn, which are causing severe pain but are not life threatening.
- Approach with caution and if the dog makes any attempt to bite, use a muzzle before beginning treatment (see page 41).
- Your treatment concerns preventing the injury from worsening and preparing the dog for transportation to the veterinarian.

3. Minor injuries or illness

- Injuries or illness such as a slight abrasion or cut come last in the order of priorities for treatment.
- Treat at home if you know how.
- Take the dog to the veterinarian if the injury worsens, for example, if signs of inflammation develop and/or the dog develops a temperature.

THE INJURED DOG

Approaching, Calming, Handling, Assessing, Lifting and Carrying

APPROACHING
• Approach an injured dog with caution as a dog that is frightened or in pain may attempt to bite.
• Before touching the dog, check for the following signs:

- The dog is conscious or unconscious (see page 15).
- The dog is bleeding (see page 61) or there is blood on the ground.
- There are obvious wounds (see page 90) or broken bones (see page 74).
- The dog's breathing is normal or laboured, rapid, shallow or absent (see page 45).
- The dog appears to be in a state of shock (see page 89).
- The dog is aggressive, most often indicated by a snarl or growl, baring of upper teeth or ears laid back.

CALMING
• Be cautious when calming an injured dog as, depending on the nature of the injury and the dog's disposition, the dog may attempt to bite if the injured area is touched.
• Talk to the dog quietly and soothingly. If there are no signs of aggression, stroke the dog whilst talking. This is a soft, calm action unlike patting which may disturb the dog and provoke an aggressive reaction.
• If the injured dog is immobile, see that the dog is in a comfortable position. If moving around excitedly, confine the dog to a small space in the company of a reassuring person.
• If the dog appears to be cold, for example, shivering

14

and shaking, then put a blanket or rug either over or around the dog's body according to the circumstances.
• If the dog appears to be excessively hot, for example, panting vigorously and rapidly, cool the dog down by using a fan or an icepack.

If the dog is unconscious and breathing

HANDLING

• Roll the dog over on to the right side with the head tilted backwards and in a position lower than the rest of the body. Advantages of this position are:

- It opens up the airway.
- It prevents the tongue obstructing the airway.
- Vomit, fluid and foreign material will drain out of the mouth.
- It makes it easier to observe and check the dog's breathing and heartbeat.

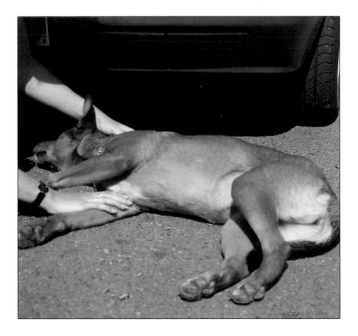

An unconscious dog should be positioned lying on the right side.

15

• Cover the dog with a blanket or towel to help maintain normal body temperature. The blanket should not restrict breathing nor make it difficult to check breathing or circulation (colour of gums and tongue, heartbeat), or other injuries.

If the dog is unconscious, not breathing, and perhaps has a blue tongue

• Apply resuscitation immediately (see page 45) and check for severe bleeding (see age 61) before making any further assessment.

If the dog is conscious and aggressive

• Make and apply a muzzle (see page 41).
• Then assess the dog's condition.
• If you cannot manage the dog, contact your veterinarian immediately.

If the dog is conscious and not aggressive

• Rub the back of your hand behind the dog's ears and then turn your hand to take a good handful of the scruff of its neck. This grip gives you good control of the dog, particularly the head.
• Then assess the dog's condition.

ASSESSING THE DOG'S CONDITION

Look at the colour of the gums

• If pale or white and there is no sign of severe external bleeding, the dog is probably suffering from shock (see page 89) or internal blood loss. Take the dog to the veterinarian immediately.
• If the gums are pink, it is a good sign that there is no major blood loss externally or internally.

Carefully run your free hand over the dog's body

• Look and feel for a wound, swelling or painful area.
• Check the movement of the limbs and note if there is pain, swelling, a grating sensation, a floppy limb irregular in appearance, or the dog itself cannot move one or more

limbs. These signs indicate that the limb, pelvis or spine may be broken (fractured) (see page 74) or the joint dislocated .

Prop the dog up on four legs and encourage the dog to walk

• If the dog flops down, walks on three legs and carries the fourth, limps, staggers, refuses to move, cries frequently as if in pain or breathes in a laboured, panting fashion, wrap the dog in a blanket for warmth and to counteract shock (see page 89). Take the dog to your veterinarian immediately.

If the dog is able to stand but reluctant to walk

• Lift the dog by hooking one arm under and around the neck and against the chest and the other under and around the abdomen.

If the dog is unable to stand or is too heavy to carry in the arms

• Improvise a stretcher by placing a towel, rug, blanket or coat on the ground next to the injured dog.
• Take the dog by the scruff of the neck in a firm grip and pull the dog onto the stretcher.
• One person takes hold of the corners of the stretcher at one end while another person holds the corners at the other end.
• Lift and carry the dog to safety nearby, then either home or to a car for transportation to a veterinary hospital.
• See page 19.

LIFTING AND CARRYING

Pink gums indicate
no major blood loss.

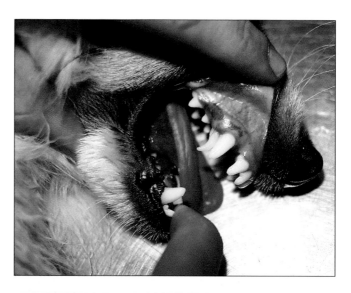

Check the movement
of the dog's limbs
for indications of
fracture, break or
dislocation.

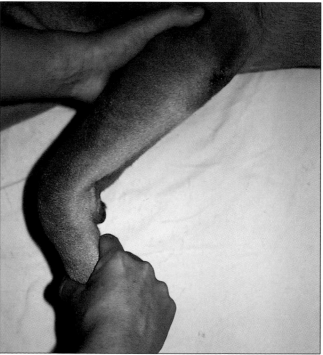

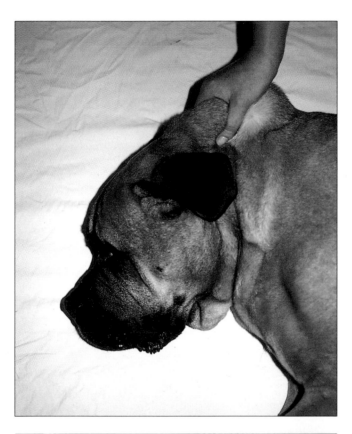

Take a handful of the scruff of the neck to gain good control over the dog.

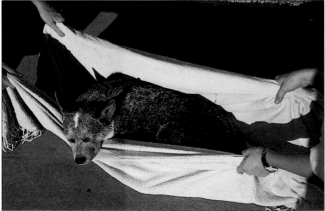

Use a blanket or similar item as a sling to lift the dog.

WHEN TO CALL YOUR VETERINARIAN

The following information may serve as a guide if you are uncertain when to call your veterinarian.

CALL IMMEDIATELY

• **Birth difficulty** No pup appears after straining for 30 minutes; if, after straining for a period of time, the bitch gives up; if part of a pup appears but nothing else appears after 20 minutes of straining.

• **Bleeding heavily** From any part of the body; will not stop. Apply pressure to stop the bleeding on the way to the veterinarian (see page 61).

• **Blood in urine** Obvious blood in urine.

• **Blood in vomit and/or severe diarrhea** Evidence of blood; putrid, fluid diarrhea.

• **Burns** Fairly extensive; or if in doubt (see page 64).

• **Choking** Appears distressed; extends head and neck; salivates; coughs; paws at the mouth (see page 65).

• **Collapse or loss of balance** Over-reaction to external stimuli; depression; staggering or knuckling over; walking in circles; down and unable to get up; general muscle tremor; rigidity; paddling movements of legs; coma.

• **Pain** Severe, continuous or spasmodic.

• **Poisoning** Chemical, snake, spider or plant. If possible, retain sample for veterinarian to identify type of poisoning (see page 80).

• **Self-mutilation** Continual uncontrollable scratching, biting, tearing at the skin; skin broken and bleeding.

• **Severe breathing distress** Gasping; noisy breathing;

blue tongue. If breathing not evident apply resuscitation (see page 45).

• **Severe injury** Severe continuous pain; severe lameness; cut with bone exposed, or puncture wound, especially eye, chest or abdomen (see page 90); fracture (see page 74); other injuries assessed as serious.

• **Straining continually** Attempting to defecate (pass a motion or stool) or urinate with little or no result.

• **Abortion (miscarriage)** Expulsion of the foetus after first three weeks of pregnancy.

CALL SAME DAY

• **Afterbirth** If retained for eight hours.

• **Appetite loss** Not eating; depressed in conjunction with other signs such as laboured breathing, diarrhea, lying down, pain.

• **Breathing difficulty** Laboured breathing; rapid and shallow breathing with or without cough.

• **Eye problems** Tears streaming down cheeks; eyelids partially or completely closed; cornea (surface of eye) cloudy, opaque or bluish-white in colour.

• **Frequent vomiting** Evident on a number of occasions; associated with some other symptom such as lethargy.

• **Frostbite and/or hypothermia** Low body temperature usually associated with sub-zero temperatures (see page 76 and/or 78).

• **Injuries** Not urgent, but liable to become infected; a cut through full thickness of skin which needs stitching; puncture wound in leg or head; acute sudden lameness.

• **Mismating** Termination of an unwanted pregnancy can be done safely and harmlessly within 72 hours after intercourse.

• **Severe diarrhea** Motion (stool) is fluid and putrid or there is abdominal pain or straining.

• **Severe itching** Biting; scratching; hair loss; skin red and inflamed.

• **Swallowed object** Better for veterinarian to assess early, rather than wait until a possible life-threatening situation develops.

• **Swelling** Hot, hard and painful or discharging.

WAIT 24 HOURS BEFORE CALLING

• **Appetite loss** Not eating; no other sign or symptom.

• **Diarrhea** Motion (stool) is semi-solid; no indication of abdominal pain; no sign of blood; no straining.

• **Itching** Moderate; no damage to the skin by self-mutilation.

• **Lameness** Ability to bear weight on leg; not affecting eating or other functions.

• **Occasional vomiting** On two or three occasions with no other symptoms.

• **Odour** Unpleasant odour other than a soiled coat.

• **Thirst** Excessive drinking, often paired with excessive urination.

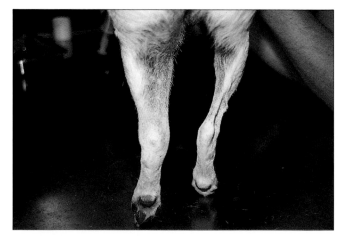

Hot, painful swelling should be checked by the veterinarian on the same day the symptoms occur.

TECHNIQUES YOU SHOULD KNOW

Bandaging

In serious, life-threatening situations, such as severe bleeding, it is more important to apply firm pressure first, with the hand or a gauze pad and bandage, and then to clean the wound later.

Steps in bandaging

• If possible, clean the wound of any debris and clip any invasive hair surrounding the wound. Cover with a cotton gauze pad or a clean handkerchief.
• Wrap a cotton gauze bandage firmly over the pad covering the wound.
• Secure the gauze bandage by wrapping an adhesive bandage firmly over it, allowing some of the adhesive bandage to stick to the hair on either side of the gauze bandage.

Types of Bandage

Adhesive

• Provides a non-slip covering difficult for the dog to remove.
• Should never be applied directly to a wound except in an emergency.
• Ideal size is 2.5cm (1in) or 7.5cm (3in) wide.
• To avoid applying it too tightly, unroll a manageable portion first before wrapping it on.

Cotton gauze

• Gauze bandages alone tend to slip and are easily torn off by the dog.
• The best type is one that adheres to itself. It does not unravel and tends to conform to the shape of the dog, and it is firmer and less bulky as a bandage.
• The end of the bandage can be secured by sticking it down with adhesive bandage. Another way is to cut the end down the middle to about 15cm (6in). Tie a knot at

the base of the two tape-like pieces to prevent further tearing and tie the tapes to secure the bandage.
• The ideal size is 2.5cm (1in) wide.

Vetwrap bandage

• A strong, self-adhering bandage which will not unravel or slip and can be used more than once.
• It is soft and conforms to that part of the dog being bandaged.
• It is used to cover a gauze bandage or dressing.
• It is not as tough as an adhesive bandage and is more easily torn and pulled off by the dog.

The dog's shape and coat of hair make it doubly difficult to apply a bandage that will stay in place. The most often bandaged areas are the abdomen, chest, ear, eye and limb.

How to Bandage

Abdomen and chest

• Apply gauze pad after cleaning the wound.
• Fix pad with strips of adhesive bandage.
• Wrap cotton gauze bandage around the body four or five times.
• Apply adhesive bandage over the gauze bandage as well as hair on either side (see page 26).

Ear

• Clean the wound and cut away any invasive hair prior to bandaging.
• Place a gauze pad over the wound and secure the pad with adhesive strips.
• To stop the dog flicking or flapping the ear, lay the ear flat on top of the head and wrap a gauze bandage two or three times over that ear, under the neck and around behind the free ear. Secure with adhesive bandage over it and the nearby hair. Carefully cut a small hole near the opening of the ear canal to allow air circulation to prevent any infection developing there (see page 27).

1. The first step in bandaging is to apply a gauze pad after cleaning the wound

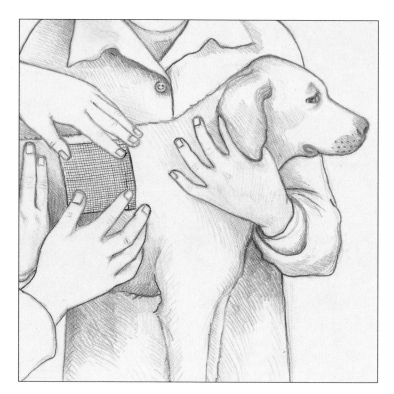

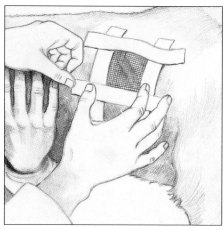

2. Fix pad with strips of adhesive.

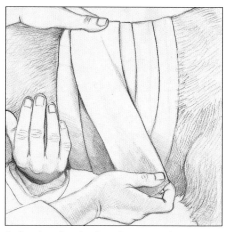

3. Apply adhesive bandage over the gauze bandage as well as hair on either side.

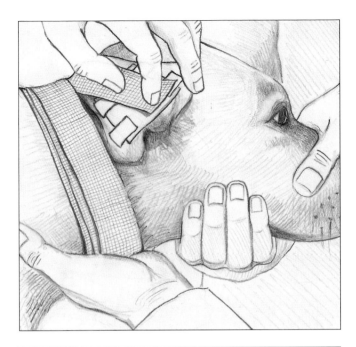

To stop the dog flicking or flapping the ear, lay the ear flat on top of the head and wrap a gauze bandage over the ear and under the neck.

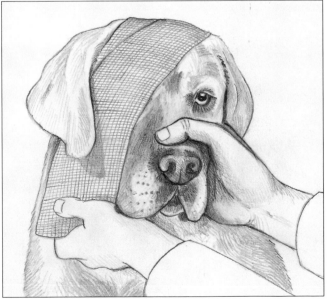

Secure a gauze pad to the eye with a gauze bandage starting behind the opposite ear and passing across the sore eye, under the jaw and back behind the ear where it began.

Eye

• Apply gauze pad to sore eye.
• Cover pad with a gauze bandage, starting behind the ear on the opposite side to the sore eye and passing it down across the sore eye, under the jaw and back behind the ear where it began. Repeat two or three turns in this direction.
• Secure by wrapping an adhesive bandage over the gauze and the nearby hair. See page 27. If the dog tries to pull or rub the bandage off, apply an Elizabethan collar (see page 32).

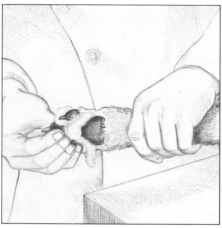

1. Clean the wound and put cottonwool (absorbent cotton) between the toes.

Foot

• Clean the wound.
• Put cottonwool (absorbent cotton) between toes.
• Apply a gauze pad to the wound.
• Wind gauze bandage around paw, up beyond the largest pad, making it more secure by twisting it to face about after every two turns.
• Secure with adhesive bandage.

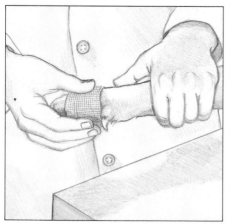

2. Apply a gauze pad to the wound.

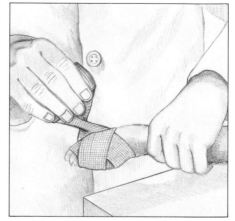

3. Wind gauze bandage around paw, making it more secure by twisting it after every two turns

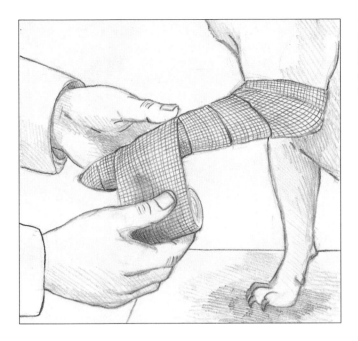

1. When bandaging a leg, wind cotton gauze bandage over a gauze pad and around the leg three or four times.

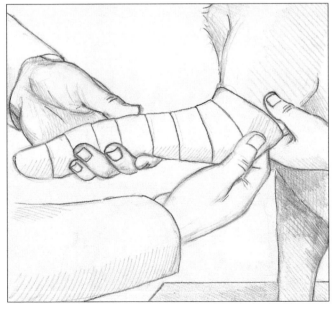

2. Secure with a similar adhesive bandage partly adhering to the dog's hair.

Leg

• Apply gauze pad to the wound after cleaning and cutting away any invasive hair.
• Wind cotton gauze bandage around the leg three or four times and secure with a similar adhesive bandage partly adhering to the dog's hair. See page 29.

Keep in mind

• Bandages should never be too tight nor too loose.
• If blood from a wound is coming through a bandage, do not remove but apply a slightly tighter adhesive bandage over it.
• If a very firm to tight bandage is on a limb for any length of time, for example, 30 minutes or more, check the limb below the bandage. If it is swollen, cold to the touch or does not react to pain when pinched, remove the bandage immediately and, if necessary, apply a new bandage less tightly.

Bleeding — How to Stop

Action

• Remain calm.
• Immobilise the dog by holding firmly.
• Apply pressure directly to the site with a clean wad of cloth or, if no cloth is available, use your hand or fingers only.
• Apply icepack to the site if the source of bleeding is inaccessible.
• See page 61 for further information on controlling bleeding.

Do not

• Dab or wipe site as this tends to promote bleeding.
• Clean site until bleeding has stopped as this might encourage fresh bleeding.

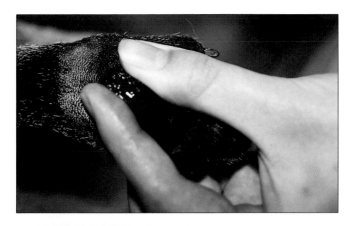

Apply pressure using finger and thumb to stop bleeding.

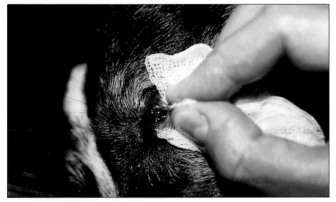

Apply pressure using a clean wad of cloth to stop bleeding.

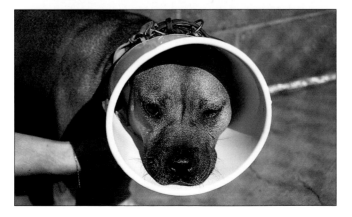

An Elizabethan collar is simple to make at home and will stop your dog from interfering with a wound or bandages.

Elizabethan Collar — Making and Fitting

Wearing an Elizabethan collar prevents a dog biting itself, pulling out stitches, chewing a plaster cast, licking a wound, tearing off a bandage or scratching the ears or face. Your veterinarian can supply you with a commercial type or you can make your own (see page 31):

• Select a suitably sized plastic bucket, that is, one that if you cut out the bottom, the head of the dog will just pass through. When it is in place the rim should protrude about 5cm (2in) beyond the dog's muzzle.
• Cut the appropriate-sized hole in the bottom of the bucket and punch six to ten evenly spaced small holes around the rim of the hole.
• Thread short lengths of string or nylon cord through each hole and tie each to make small loops so that the dog's collar can be passed through each one.
• Put the bucket over the dog's head and fasten the collar firmly so that the bucket is anchored to the dog's neck.

Caution

• Keep the dog confined or if going for a walk, keep the dog on a lead as the Elizabethan collar limits the dog's field of vision.
• An alternative to taking off the collar when the dog is feeding is to leave the collar on and hold the food or water bowl to the dog's mouth.

Heartbeat and Pulse — How to Check

• The normal pulse of the dog varies according to breed, age, weight, and so on.
• The normal pulse rate ranges from 80 to 120 beats per minute.
• The pulse is a reflection of the heartbeat; it is an indicator of blood circulation.

Where to Feel the Pulse

• To obtain a correct reading, the dog must be calm.
• Place a finger (not the thumb) on the inside of the thigh near the groin and feel gently in the area for a pulse from the artery just under the skin (see page 34).

Where to Feel the Heartbeat

• The heartbeat is best located behind the left elbow between the third and sixth rib.
• The beat can be observed as a regular slight movement of the chest wall on the left side in the area where the heart is located (see page 34).

Heartbeat as a Guide

• If the heartbeat is an average 80 to 120 beats per minute, the circulation system is normal.
• If the heartbeat is outside the average, see your veterinarian.

No Heartbeat or Pulse

• Apply the cardiac compression technique immediately (see page 45).

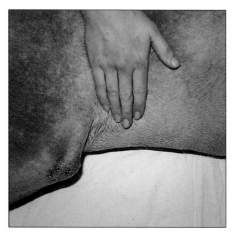

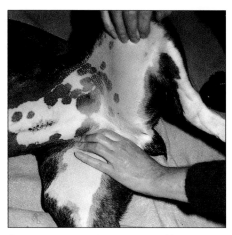

Feel for the heartbeat behind the left elbow between the third and sixth rib.

Check the pulse by placing a finger on the inside of the thigh near the groin.

Leg Fracture — Robert Jones Bandage Technique

The Robert Jones Bandage Technique described below gives good immobilisation and support and does not interfere with circulation:

• Evenly wrap layers of cottonwool (absorbent cotton) around the fractured limb well above and below as well as over the site of the fracture.

• Compress the layers of cottonwool (absorbent cotton) by very firmly wrapping several rolls of gauze bandage over them.

• Finally, wrap a number of layers of adhesive bandage around the gauze bandage and nearby hair.

• Pinch the dog's toes to see that circulation has not been interfered with. If the dog reacts by pulling the foot away or crying, the pain sensation indicates good circulation.

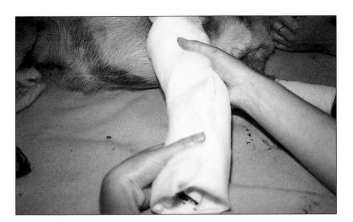

1. The Robert Jones Bandage Technique begins with wrapping layers of cottonwool (absorbent cotton) around the fractured limb.

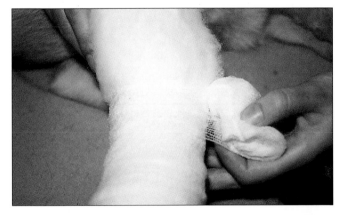

2. Compress the cottonwool (absorbent cotton) by firmly wrapping several layers of gauze bandage over them.

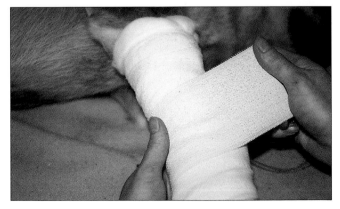

3. Finally, wrap a number of layers of adhesive bandage around the gauze bandage and nearby hair.

Medicine — How to Administer

Medicines come in many forms: tablet, capsule, powder, granule, liquid, paste, ointment, drops or injection. How the medicine is to be given and in what form depends on such factors as its type and palatability, the condition and temperament of the dog, and the owner's temperament. Some tablets, powders and granules are flavoured to make them palatable. This type can be handfed to the dog or mixed thoroughly with the dog's food. If it is mixed with the food, check the food bowl to make sure the dog has eaten it. Dogs are very suspicious of any foreign materials in their food and some will sort it out or reject their food completely.

If your dog's medicine is in the form of unpalatable tablets you can choose one of several methods to administer it: with the fingers; with a pill popper; or with a spoon. With each of these methods it is essential to know how to open a dog's mouth (see also page 39).

How to Open a Dog's Mouth

• Put the dog in a small room, for example, the laundry or utility room. If the dog is small, use a table.
• If the dog is restless, get an assistant to hold the dog firmly while you open the mouth in one quick movement.
• With one hand grasp the upper jaw between your fingers and thumb.
• Tilt the dog's head back so that it is looking toward the ceiling.
• Using the middle finger of your other hand, press the front of the lower jaw down to open the mouth wider but not too wide as the dog will become distressed.

Giving a Tablet with the Fingers

• Open the dog's mouth, place the tablet, held between the thumb and index finger, over the back of the dog's tongue. It may be necessary to quickly push the tablet

further over the back of the tongue (see page 39).
• Remove your finger quickly before the dog closes its mouth.
• Keep the dog's head tilted back and massage the throat to stimulate swallowing. When the dog licks the upper lip with the tongue, the pill has been swallowed.

Caution

• Keep the dog's head tilted back or it will be difficult to drop the tablet over the back of the tongue.
• Ensure the tablet is over the back of the tongue or the dog will spit it out.

• Put the tablet in the pill popper, a device or instrument used to place a tablet over the back of the dog's tongue.
• Open the dog's mouth (see page 36).
• Quickly and smoothly place the end of the pill popper into the back of the dog's mouth.
• Press the plunger to release the tablet over the back of the tongue.
• Withdraw the popper, keep the head tilted back and rub the dog's throat to stimulate swallowing.

Giving a Tablet with a Pill Popper

• Place the tablet in the spoon.
• Open the dog's mouth (see page 36).
• Insert the spoon so that it is pressing down on the front of the lower jaw.
• Tip the tablet over the back of the tongue.
• Withdraw the spoon, keep the head tilted back and rub the dog's throat to stimulate swallowing.

Giving a Tablet with a Spoon

• Open the dog's mouth with one hand and tilt the head back slightly (see page 36 and 39).
• Holding a syringe or eye-dropper in the other hand, slowly dribble the liquid onto the back of the tongue.
• If the dog does not swallow, tilt the head a little more and dribble more liquid onto the back of the tongue.

Administering Liquids — Method 1

Caution

• If the dog coughs and splutters, the liquid may be flowing into the windpipe. Correct by not tilting the head so far back.

Administering Liquids — Method 2

• Tilt the dog's head back.
• Hook your finger into the corner of the dog's mouth and pull out the cheek slightly to form a pouch.
• Slowly dribble the liquid from the syringe or eye-dropper into the pouch allowing sufficient time for the dog to swallow.

Caution

• If the liquid is unpleasant the dog may salivate profusely, causing saliva and the liquid to dribble out of the mouth. Re-adminster approximately the same amount of liquid as was dribbled. If concerned about a possible overdose, consult your veterinarian.

Administering a Paste

• Open the dog's mouth (see page 36).
• Apply the paste, which usually comes in a syringe, to the dog's tongue. The paste will adhere to the tongue and be swallowed.

Caution

• If the paste is unpalatable the dog will salivate, causing a paste and saliva to pour from the mouth. Re-adminster approximately the same amount of paste as was dribbled. If concerned about an overdose, consult your veterinarian.

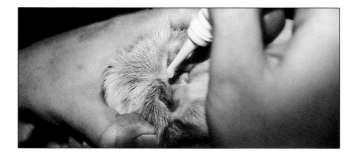

To administer ear drops, hold the ear tip with your thumb and index finger, pulling towards the other ear.

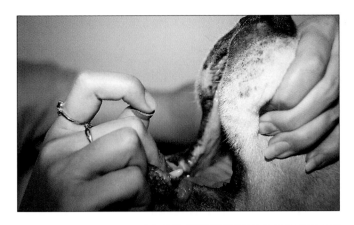

Grasp the upper jaw between fingers and thumb and tilt back the dog's head to administer a tablet with your fingers.

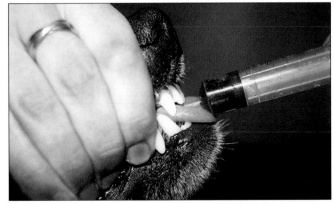

Use a syringe to slowly dribble liquid on to the back of the dog's tongue.

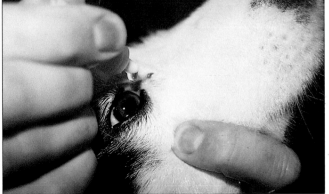

When adminstering eye drops keep the head tilted.

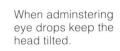

Administering Ear Drops

- Get an assistant to hold the dog firmly while you administer the drops.
- Take hold of the ear tip with your thumb and index finger, pulling it toward the opposite ear. This opens up the affected ear and makes the opening of the ear canal obvious (see page 38).
- Squeeze four to six drops into the canal.
- Continue to hold the ear and the head firmly, otherwise the dog will shake the head vigorously and spray the drops everywhere.
- With your free hand gently massage below the ear to work the drops down the ear canal.
- If the dog is fidgety do not worry to count the drops, just put the nozzle of the container in the ear canal and give it a squirt. Stop when you see the drops starting to well up out of the ear canal.

Administering Eye Drops

- Get an assistant to hold the dog firmly and tilt its head slightly back.
- Gently hold the eyelids apart with your thumb and index finger.
- Administer two drops on each eyeball. Keep the head tilted for about 20 seconds or the eyedrops will roll out and be wasted (see page 39).

Administering Eye Ointment

- Get an assistant to hold the dog firmly while you administer the medication.
- With your thumb, pull either the lower lid down or the upper lid up and lay a strip of ointment inside the lid along its full length.
- Close the eyelid. The ointment will melt forming a film over eyeball and conjunctiva.

Injections

If other methods of administering medicine are impossible because of the dog's temperament or condition, an injection may be the only alternative. This is best left to the veterinarian.

Muzzle — Making and Applying

When in pain, a normally placid dog may bite. A muzzle allows you to handle the dog without fear of being bitten.
• Take a piece of material about 1m (3ft) long, such as a gauze bandage, nylon stocking or neck tie.
• Hold both ends of the material, and make a closed loop with a half knot.
• Whilst talking soothingly to try to calm the dog, slip the loop over the dog's muzzle and draw tightly so that the half knot is on the top of the dog's nose.
• Make another closed loop with a half knot, and slip it around the dog's muzzle but with the half knot under the lower jaw.
• Complete the muzzle by bringing the two ends, one each side, above the dog's neck and tying them in a tight bow behind the dog's ears for quick release (see page 42).

Orphan Puppy — How to Feed

When your puppy must be handfed your veterinarian can supply you with a commercial milk substitute or you can make up your own.

• Two formulas for substitute milk are:
- One cup of evaporated or powdered milk mixed with boiled water and made up to double the strength recommended on the container for babies. Mix in one egg yolk and one teaspoon of glucose substitute.
- Half a cup of cow's milk. Mix in one egg yolk and one teaspoon of glucose substitute.

• The faeces will give you an indication as to whether the milk substitute you are using is too rich. If the puppy has diarrhea, dilute the milk substitute. If diarrhea continues, consult your veterinarian.

Do you know?

Sometimes a puppy has to be handfed because its mother died at birth, or has no milk or rejects the puppy. Or, the puppy itself, because of weakness or some other reason, is unable to suckle.

1. To construct a muzzle, make a closed loop with a half knot and slip over the dog's nose.

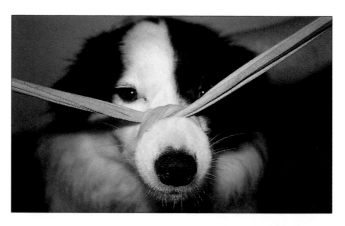

2. Make another closed loop with a half knot and pull tightly so the half knot is under the jaw.

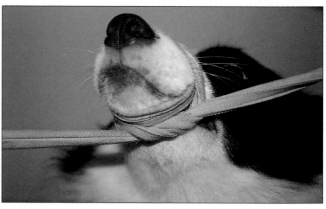

3. Complete the muzzle by tying a tight bow behind the dog's ears.

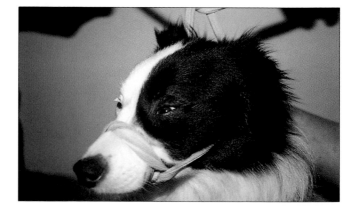

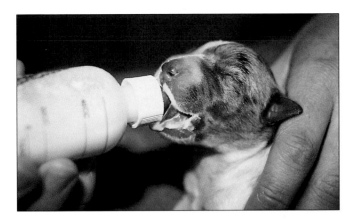

Move the teat in and out of the mouth when bottle feeding a puppy.

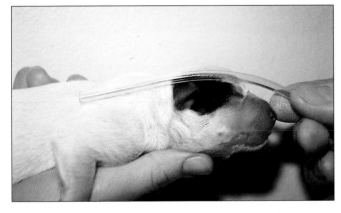

1. When stomach tube feeding, measure the length of a soft, plastic tube from the puppy's mouth to a point two-thirds along the ribcage.

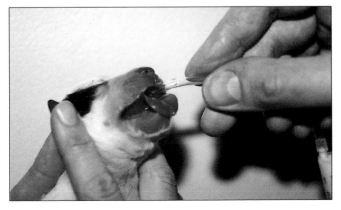

2. Insert the tube gently but firmly over the back of the tongue and into the food pipe.

• If possible, express the colostrum (first milk) from the mother's nipples and give it to the orphan puppy either with the substitute milk or separately.
• Warm the milk to body temperature before feeding.

Feeding Times

• Feed the puppy every two hours in the first week of life, giving about 5ml (1 teaspoon) of milk substitute at each feed. This amount can vary according to individual demand.
• Thereafter, gradually decrease the frequency of feeding and increase the amount of milk substitute.
• By the time the puppy is two weeks old, four-hourly feeding is sufficient.

Bottle Feeding

• Hold the puppy firmly, elevate the head slightly and insert the teat into the pup's mouth.
• Move the teat in and out of the mouth and express a small amount of milk to encourage the puppy to suck.

Stomach Tube Feeding

• You will need a soft plastic tube 3mm (0.1 in) in diameter and 15cm (6in) long, attached to a syringe.
• Measure the distance on the tube from the puppy's mouth to a point two-thirds along the ribcage.
• Mark the distance on the tube to indicate how far the tube has to be inserted via the puppy's mouth to reach the stomach.
• Insert the tube gently but firmly and with great care, pushing it over the back of the tongue into the food pipe (esophagus), until it reaches the stomach.
• Ask your veterinarian to give you a demonstration or enlist the help of an experienced breeder (see page 43).

Resuscitation — Breathing (Mouth-to-nose) and Heartbeat (Cardiac Compression)

Check the dog's mouth or nose for any foreign body or food obstructing the airway. If an obstruction is present use one of the following methods to remove it:

• **Small dog** Hold the dog upside down by the hind legs and shake vigorously five or six times.

• **Large dog** Lay the dog on the side and, if necessary, use long-nosed pliers to clear any solid obstruction in the mouth.

To perform mouth-to-nose resuscitation

• Lay the dog on the right side, with head back and mouth closed (see page 46).
• Place a cloth, for example, a handkerchief, over the dog's nose (for cosmetic reasons only).
• Place your open mouth over the dog's nose and breathe into it quickly five or six times. For a young puppy with a small lung capacity, the breaths are short and shallow; for a large dog, the breaths are longer and deeper.
• If breathing is restored, keep the dog under observation.
• If breathing is not restored, apply mouth-to-nose resuscitation at the rate of one breath every three seconds, that is, 20 breaths per minute.
• Continue to repeat until breathing is restored. If it is, keep the dog under observation.
• If breathing is not restored after 10 minutes, the gums and tongue are blue, the pupils are dilated and there is no blinking when the surface of the eye is touched, you can presume the dog is dead.

If Breathing has Stopped

Do you know?

• The average dog's breathing rate is 20 breaths per minute.
• The average dog's heartbeat (pulse rate) is 80 to 120 beats per minute.
• Immediate, yet calm, treatment is essential in resuscitation.

1. Hold the dog's mouth closed for resuscitation.

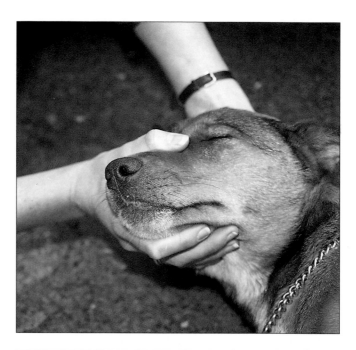

2. Place your open mouth over the dog's nose and breathe into it quickly five or six times. You can cover the nose with a cloth, for example, a handkerchief.

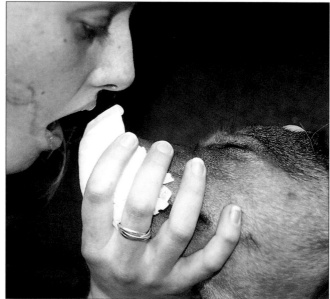

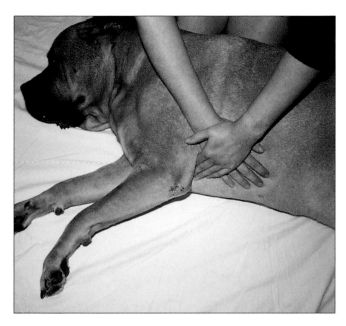

Cardiac compresssion
for a large dog,
showing position
of hands.

• Lay the dog on the right side.
• If a small dog or puppy, with one hand place your
thumb on one side of the chest and your fingers on the
other in the area between the third and sixth ribs just
below the left elbow.
• If a large dog, place the heel of the hand over the area
between the third and sixth ribs just below the left
elbow.
• The force applied to the heart area in cardiac
compression varies according to the size of the dog, from
fingertip compression for a young puppy to heel-of-the-
hand compression for a large dog.
• Give 10 quick compressions. If the heartbeat and pulse
are restored, keep the dog under observation.
• If the heartbeat and pulse are not restored, continue to
apply cardiac compression in cycles of 10 at the rate of
10 cycles per minute, that is about 10 compressions
every six seconds. When the heartbeat and pulse are
restored, keep the dog under observation.

If Heartbeat (Pulse) has Stopped

• If there is no sign of heartbeat and pulse after 10 minutes, the gums and tongue are blue, the pupils are dilated and there is no blinking when the surface of the eye is touched, you can presume the dog is dead.

If Breathing and Heartbeat (Pulse) have Stopped

• If there are two people present: one person gives about 10 cardiac compressions followed by the second person giving two mouth-to-nose expired air breaths. Repeat this synchronised sequence at about the rate of 10 per minute, that is about one sequence every six seconds.
• If one person is present: give 10 cardiac compressions followed by two mouth-to-nose expired air breaths. Repeat this sequence at the rate of about 10 cycles per minute, that is about one sequence every six seconds.

Temperature — How to Check

The normal temperature for a dog ranges between 37.8°C (100°F) and 39.2°C (102.5°F). If your dog's temperature remains outside that range see your veterinarian, as the dog probably has an infection or some other illness.

Action

• An ordinary household thermometer may be used.
• Shake the mercury down to below 37.8°C (100°F) and smear the thermometer with a non-irritant lubricant, such as Vaseline.
• Insert it into the dog's anus to about 5cm (2in) with the bulb resting against the rectal wall.
• Withdraw the thermometer after one to two minutes and check the reading.
• Wipe thermometer clean with disinfectant, and store in a suitable container.
• Wash hands thoroughly.

Umbilical Cord —
How to Sever and Treat

• The bitch often breaks the umbilical cord when she is licking, pulling and tearing at the foetal membrane to free the pup from it.
• If the umbilical cord is not broken, wait five to 10 minutes before severing it; otherwise, the pup may suffer brain damage.

Action

• To prevent bleeding, apply a ligature by tightly tying thread soaked in disinfectant around the umbilical cord about 2cm ($^3/_4$in) from the pup's body (see page 54).
• Cut the cord with scissors soaked in disinfectant 1cm ($^1/_3$in) from the ligature, on the placental side. Or, break the cord with your fingers.
• Swab the cut end with tincture of iodine.

Caution

• Premature breaking of the cord may deprive the puppy of its maximum blood supply, thus starving the brain of oxygen and causing subsequent damage.
• If the end of the cord is bleeding when severed by the bitch, control the haemorrhage by tying the cord off with disinfected thread.

FIRST AID FOR INJURIES AND ILLNESS

Abscess

• An abscess is a collection of pus, circumscribed in a sac, and enclosed within the tissues of the body.
• Abscesses may be due to a foreign body, such as a nail or grass seed, entering the body and setting up an infection, or to bacteria lodging in an organ. The latter type of abscess occurs after a generalised infection, in which case the abscess might appear on the liver or lungs.

Signs

• Pain felt by dog when touched at the site of the abscess.
• The dog may be lethargic, without an appetite and/or have a temperature.
• The abscess is at first a hard lump which softens as it matures and finally may burst.
• A puncture wound from a bite or a sharp foreign body are common causes.

Action

• Cut away surrounding hair and bathe the wound with a cloth or cottonwool (absorbent cotton) soaked in hot water for 10 minutes twice daily.
• If a puncture wound is obvious, clean with iodine-based scrub or 3% hydrogen peroxide. Remove any foreign body that may be embedded in the wound.
• If the abscess bursts, clean as suggested and gently squeeze out any evident discharge.
• If the abscess does not burst, the veterinarian will open the abscess, drain out the pus and administer antibiotics.
• If the abscess continues to drain after being opened, it should be irrigated twice daily using a syringe containing 3% hydrogen peroxide.

Birth Problems

• In rendering First Aid at a birth scene, make sure your hands have been scrubbed with a non-irritant antiseptic and that you are wearing surgical gloves if available.
• If you cannot give the necessary First Aid, get in touch with your veterinarian immediately.

If the pup is born in its amnion sac (membrane)

• The bitch ruptures it with her teeth to release the puppy, licks the puppy to clean it and chews through the umbilical cord if it is not broken. If the bitch neglects to do so, you must do it, especially cleaning the puppy's airways (nose and mouth) of any membrane and mucus so that it can breathe. See page 49 for breaking of the umbilical cord.

Puppy's head presented at the vulva but the bitch cannot expel it

• Scrub your hands and the area around the bitch's anus and vulva with a non-irritant antiseptic.
• If the membranes are intact, break them with your fingers to clear the puppy's nose and mouth so that breathing is possible.
• Get a good grip of the puppy by removing any visible membrane and, with a piece of clean towelling material in your hand, take hold of the puppy around the shoulder area.
• Slowly pull outward and downward. If the puppy will not budge, a twist to the left or right in conjunction with pulling will often bring about success. Always pull as the bitch is having a contraction.

One leg presented at the vulva

• Put your finger into the vagina and feel for the other leg. Pull it outward, then proceed to deliver the pup.

Do you know?

• Puppies are usually born 10 to 30 minutes apart.
• All the puppies are usually born over a period of three to six hours although this can vary.
• The normal presentation of the newborn puppy at the vulva is head first.

The large abscess under this dog's jaw may have been caused by a puncture wound from a bite or a sharp foreign body.

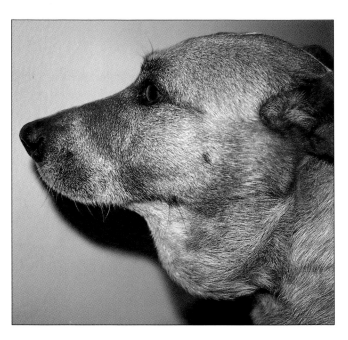

Before severing an umbilical cord, prevent bleeding by tying the cord with disinfected thread. See page 49.

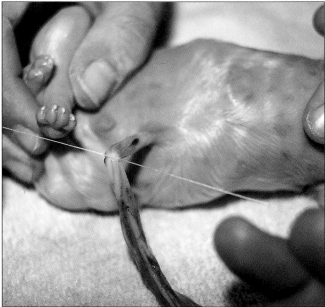

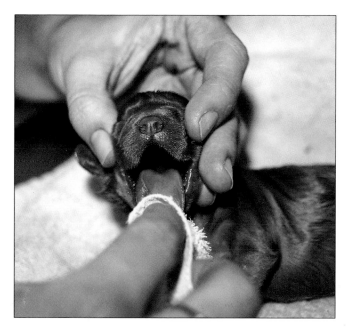

Wipe away any placental membrane or mucus from the newborn puppy's mouth to allow breathing.

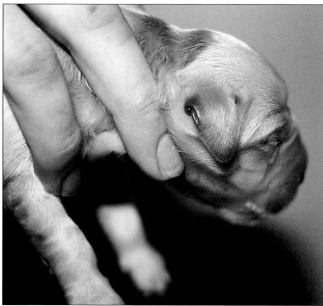

The newborn puppy should be gripped in this manner while attempting to restore breathing. See page 56.

Hindquarters presented at the vulva

• Take hold of the pup in the region of the hips.
Pull outward and downward as the bitch is having
a contraction.

Caution

• Avoid squeezing the abdomen as this can cause serious
damage.

No puppy present at the vulva

Call your veterinarian if:
- The bitch has been straining for more than 30 minutes
and no pup appears.
- There are no obvious contractions and the bitch is
distressed, continually getting up and down, looking at
her flanks and crying.
- After 30 minutes of obvious straining and contractions,
the bitch appears to give up and her efforts are weak and
less frequent.

Newborn puppy not breathing

• Check the airways to see that they are clear. If
necessary, wipe away any placental membranes or mucus
that may be blocking the puppy's nostrils or mouth.
• Lay the puppy, with the head lower than the rest of the
body, on a towel wrapped around a hot water bottle (not
too hot). Warmth is very important and the head-down
position allows the blood to flow more freely to the
brain.
• Rub the puppy's chest briskly with a towel to stimulate
breathing.
• If the puppy is still not breathing gently massage the
chest, positioned between your thumb and fingers.
• If still no sign of breathing, grip the puppy safely
cradled in your hand with the head protruding from
between your index and middle fingers. Raise the held
puppy above your head and proceed with an action as if

you were going to throw the pup to the ground. Repeat this action four or five times to rid the nose and mouth of any mucus and stimulate circulation (see page 55).
• Finally, if the puppy is still not breathing, apply mouth-to-nose resuscitation (see page 45). A newborn puppy has only a small lung capacity so use short, shallow breaths to avoid stretching or rupturing the lungs.

Afterbirth not expelled

• Afterbirth is normally expelled with the birth of each pup or immediately after. Often the bitch will eat the afterbirth, so it may not be seen. If the afterbirth(s) is (are) not expelled within eight hours after the last pup is born, take the following action:

- If the retained afterbirth is obvious, remove it by manually pulling on it with firm, even tension.
- If this fails or the retained afterbirth is not obvious, contact your veterinarian.

Bites and Stings

DOG BITE

• Dogs inflict puncture wounds with their canine teeth when fighting.
• The usual site of puncture wounds is the neck, limbs or back.
• A puncture wound may look neat and clean on the surface but tissue under the skin can be badly torn and infected.

Signs

• A painful spot and/or blood matted in the hair.

Action

• Carefully clip the hair away from the hole.
• Clean the area with 3% hydrogen peroxide and dab the wound with tincture of iodine.

• If the puncture wound appears to penetrate through the skin into the underlying tissues, take your dog to your veterinarian who will administer antibiotics and, if necessary, provide drainage.

Caution

• Some types of puncture wounds may lead to an abscess (see page 52) or serious infection.

SNAKE BITE
Signs

• The dog is stunned, often slobbering from the mouth.
• The dog has staring, unblinking eyes.
• There is little limb movement.
• The dog may be lying on the side or chest.
• You can tell whether your dog has been bitten by a poisonous or non-poisonous snake by the bite mark. Poisonous snakes leave two fang marks (puncture wounds), the non-poisonous leave a row of small teeth marks.

Action

If the dog has been bitten on a leg

• Calm the dog.
• Apply a broad bandage with firm pressure over the fang marks and about 5cm (2in) either side of them.

If the dog has been bitten in an area that may be difficult to bandage

• Calm the dog.
• Apply ice to the site to constrict blood vessels.
• Seek veterinary help immediately.

Caution

• *Do not* apply a tourniquet as it may aggravate the problem.
• *Do not* cut the skin at the bite site as it will increase blood flow and spread of poison.

Do you know?

• Usually you do not see your dog being bitten by a snake, so know the signs.
• If you do see the snake, visualise a good description of it for the veterinarian as there are several different types of antivenene.

• An early sign is a change in the dog's voice to a croaky, husky bark.
• If the tick is about the dog's face, it may cause paralysis of eyelids or lip on the side where the tick is located.
• Pupils are dilated. The tongue may poke out of the mouth and the dog may vomit.
• Paralysis progresses to hind limbs and chest when a further sign will be grunting, distressed breathing.
• Paralysis of chest muscles leads to death by suffocation.

Action

• Hold the hair away from the tick so that you can see where the head is embedded in the skin.
• Grasp tick with tweezers as close to its embedded head as possible and pull it out.
• If part of the head is left in the skin do not worry, but dab with antiseptic.

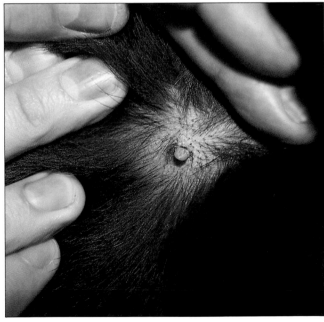

Hold hair away from the tick to reveal where the head is embedded.

Do you know?

• Only the adult female tick attaches itself to the dog and in four to six days will poison it.
• The adult female tick, oval in shape, varies in colour from grey to blue to brown. It varies in size from 2mm ($\frac{1}{8}$in) to 8mm ($\frac{1}{3}$in) depending on its engorgement with blood.

Caution

• If at any time the dog shows sign(s) of tick poisoning, take it to your veterinarian for anti-tick serum and observation.

Prevention

• Ticks are active in late spring and early summer and it is best to keep your dog away from areas of heavy plant growth and long grass at this time. Dogs should be checked for ticks daily during this period.
• Keep in mind that 80 per cent of ticks found are on the dog's head and neck; the remaining 20 per cent are found on any part of the dog.
• Rinse the dog each week in an insecticidal solution.
• Clip long-haired dogs in spring. Ticks do not attach themselves as readily to short-haired dogs and are easier to find.

UNIDENTIFIED BITE OR STING

The active dog, searching about in the garden with its nose and forelimbs, may be bitten or stung by an insect such as a bee, by a spider, or by some plant to which it is allergic.

Signs

Signs will vary but may include:

• Sudden pain and yelping.
• Rapid swelling or welts on face or paw, perhaps with inflammation.
• The dog scratching or biting the affected area.

Action

Check the site where the incident occurred. It may help you to find the cause and:

• If a bee, remove the sting and apply a cold compress or soothing lotion, for example, calamine.
• If a spider, identify it and if poisonous take the dog to your veterinarian.
• If swelling is extensive, or the dog appears distressed or in a state of shock, seek veterinary advice.

Do you know?

• There are no poisonous spiders in the UK.

Bleeding

To control the bleeding

- Remain calm.
- Immobilise the dog by holding firmly.
- Apply pressure directly to the site or apply an icepack (for example, ice in a towel) if the site is inaccessible.
- Apply bandage firmly to the site.

Caution

- *Do not* dab, wipe or attempt to clean the site until after the bleeding stops as these tend to promote bleeding.

If blood is oozing slowly

- Apply clean gauze pad to the wound and direct pressure on it with fingers.
- After 10 seconds, remove pressure and gauze pad to evaluate wound.
- If bleeding recommences, reapply gauze pad and finger pressure for a longer time, about 20 seconds.

If blood is flowing freely

- Apply gauze pad to wound and heavy, direct pressure with clean fingers or hand for about 30 seconds.
- Over the gauze pad wrap firmly but not too tightly a 7.5cm (3in) wide adhesive bandage.
- Leave bandage in place for 30 minutes then remove to evaluate wound.
- If bleeding recommences, reapply pressure bandage.

If blood is bright red, spurting with pulsating action

- This is a sign of arterial bleeding.
- With gauze pad in hand, apply heavy pressure to site for about 30 seconds.

• Wrap 7.5cm (3in) adhesive bandage tightly around gauze pad on site.
• Leave bandage in place, keep dog immobilised, preferably wrapped in a blanket, and take the dog to the veterinarian.
• If blood oozing or running through the bandage, do not remove, but apply another adhesive bandage more tightly over the top of it.

If blood is coming from an inaccessible area, for example, inside nose

Wrapping a dog in a blanket is an effective form of immobilisation.

• Apply cold in the form of an icepack and keep the dog immobilised.

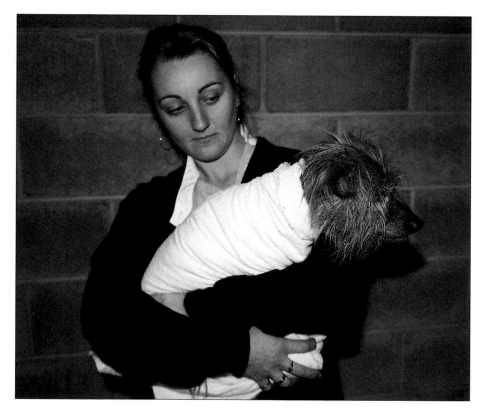

Caution

• The dog may bleed to death if you panic and hesitate.
• Keep the dog still, as movement will accelerate the bleeding. The ideal is for one person to immobilise the dog while another person controls the bleeding.
• When a pressure bandage is left on a limb for 30 minutes, always check the limb below the bandage for swelling, coldness, or no reaction to pain if pinched. If any of these signs is evident, release bandage and reapply not so firmly.
• Tourniquets are not recommended. They are often difficult to apply and if applied incorrectly, they may accentuate rather than retard bleeding.

Bloat (Gastric Dilation)

Signs

• Attempting to vomit.
• Severe abdominal pain.
• Bloated stomach. The gas-filled stomach gives off a drum-like sound when tapped with the fingers.
• Refusing to move.
• Salivating and/or panting.
• Initially excited and distressed then, as shock sets in, depressed.

Action

• *This is an emergency situation and a life-threatening illness. Take the dog to your veterinarian immediately.*

Prevention

• Feed the dog three to four small meals per day.
• Do not feed dry food to susceptible breeds of dogs. Add water to the dry food to moisten it thoroughly.
• Do not give the dog bones.
• Do not allow the dog to scavenge.
• Avoid exciting or exercising the dog before and after meals.

Do you know?

• Bloat occurs more frequently in deep-chested dogs such as Great Danes and Basset Hounds.

• Bloat may be caused by rapidly eating large volumes of food (often dry), by eating bones or foreign material such as manure or by drinking large volumes of water. These possible causes may be associated with too much exercise or excitement before or after eating and drinking.

Burns

CHEMICAL BURN

Many household products such as chlorine can cause burns, mostly to the skin and sometimes internally.

Action

• If on skin, wash thoroughly by hosing or pouring copious amounts of water on the dog for about five minutes, then gently wash the area with soap and water. Rinse thoroughly.
• If ingested, encourage the dog to drink copious amounts of water. If the dog refuses, use a syringe or gently running water from the hose to rinse the dog's mouth, thereby stimulating drinking. In the case of acid, sodium bicarbonate solution is used as an alternative to neutralise the acid.
• Take the dog to your veterinarian.

ELECTRICAL BURN

The main risk is puppies or playful dogs biting a moving electrical lead attached to, for instance, an iron or lawn mower, or a blow-drier falling into the bathtub while the dog is being washed.

Action

• Turn the power off at the switch.
• If unable to get to the switch, use a dry wooden or plastic stick to flick the plug out of the socket and to push the dog away from the source of the electricity.
• Check breathing and heartbeat (see page 33). If necessary, apply resuscitation (see page 45).
• Take the dog to your veterinarian.

• First-degree burns are the least serious; signs are various degrees of reddened skin.
• Second-degree burns are characterised by reddening of the skin with the formation of blisters.
• Third-degree burns are the most serious and are characterised by the full thickness of the skin and underlying tissues being destroyed.
• Extensive second- and third-degree burns are associated with shock, fluid loss (dehydration) and infection.

HEAT BURN
Signs

• Immediately run cold water on the burn from a hose, tap or shower; or if ice is readily available, apply it for 10 to 15 minutes; or immerse the burnt area in a basin filled with water and ice.
• Dry the area by dabbing gently. Do not rub as you may break the delicate surface.
• In the case of a second- or third-degree burn, protect the wound by covering it gently with a gauze pad or clean handkerchief held in place with a light adhesive bandage. Do not use cottonwool (absorbent cotton) because it will adhere to the surface of the burn.
• Deep or extensive burns require quick veterinary attention.

Action

Do you know?

• The burn may be fatal if more than 50% of the dog's skin is affected

Choking

• Attempting to vomit.
• Mouth open and the dog does not appear able to close it.
• Saliva dribbling from the mouth.
• Clawing of the mouth with the front paws.

Signs

• If breathing reasonably freely, take the dog to your veterinarian immediately.
• If the dog is on the verge of collapsing and the tongue is blue:

Action

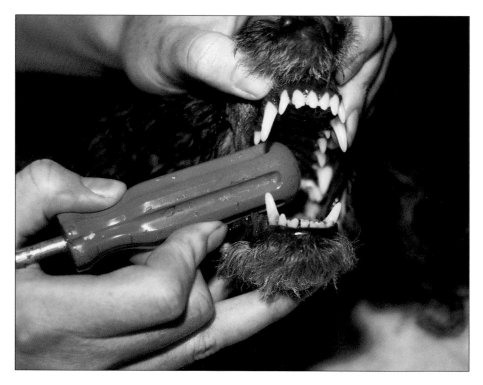

A screwdriver handle can be used to keep a dog's mouth open if choking.

- Wedge something, such as the handle of a screwdriver, between the molar teeth on one side of the dog's mouth to keep it open.
- Inspect the back of the throat, roof of the mouth and between the teeth for a foreign body.
- Pull the tongue out carefully to avoid being bitten. This may reveal a foreign body over the back of the tongue.
– Use long-nosed pliers or, if the dog cannot close the mouth, use your finger(s) to lever the foreign body out.

• If you are unable to remove the foreign body by the above method, and you can lift the dog, hold the dog upside down by the hind legs. Shake the dog vigorously to dislodge the foreign body and clear the airway.
• If the dog is not breathing, give mouth-to-nose resuscitation (see page 45).

Conjunctivitis

• The conjunctiva is the membrane lining the inside of the eyelids.
• Conjunctivitis is inflammation and/or infection of the conjunctiva.
• Puppies' eyes open seven to ten days after birth. If an infection of the conjunctiva is present, it is usually noticed at that time.

Signs

• The dog's eyelids are stuck together.
• Pus oozes from the corner of the eyelids.
• Dry pus adheres to the edges of the eyelids.

Action

• Bathe the eyelids in warm water and gently part them if stuck together; in the case of a young puppy, do not pull the eyelids apart too abruptly as you may damage the rims.
• Wipe away any discharge adhering to the eyelashes or eyelids while bathing them. This helps to prevent them sealing together again.
• Keep the dog out of the wind and direct sunlight.
• If the discharge from the dog's eye is heavy or continuous, see your veterinarian who will prescribe an appropriate eye ointment.

Caution

• There are numerous eye ointments, each of which has a specific purpose. Eye ointments should not be used indiscriminately for conjunctivitis as the wrong kind can worsen certain conditions. For example, if ulceration of the cornea (the surface of the eyeball) is incorrectly treated, the result may be blindness or a damaged eye.

Diabetic Emergency (Insulin Overdose)

An overdose of insulin causes hypoglycaemia, that is, a low blood sugar level, that could result in convulsions, coma and possibly death.

Action for Low Blood Sugar Level Due to Insulin Overdose

• If the dog is conscious but not coordinated enough to eat, carefully give through the mouth with a syringe large amounts of sugar dissolved in water, or honey, maple syrup, etc.
• If the dog can eat give canned or dried food, or cakes, biscuits, or any food high in sugar.
• Seek veterinary help.
• Once stabilised, your veterinarian will supply you with sticks to test the urine sugar level and needles, syringes and insulin to maintain the correct sugar level.

Diarrhea

Signs

• The dog defecates more frequently, and the faeces are of a porridge or fluid-like consistency, often with a very offensive odour.

Action

• Do not feed the dog for 24 hours but provide drinking water.
• If the dog has not passed a motion (stool) or the motion appears firmer, offer a small amount (a quarter of the normal daily food intake) of steamed chicken or lean, grilled meat.
• Exclude dairy products and fat from the diet until the dog has fully recovered.
• After three to four days of normal motion, slowly return the dog to a normal diet.

• If the diarrhea persists for more than 24 hours, there is blood in the motion, the dog is lethargic, vomits, or appears to have a loss of appetite, take the dog and a specimen of the faeces to your veterinarian for examination.

Drowning

Action

• Quickly remove the dog from the water.
• If breathing, hold the dog upside down by the hind legs. If too heavy, place the dog in a position where the head is lower than the chest. This action helps to drain water from the lungs.
• If the dog's breathing or heart (pulse) has stopped (see page 33), apply resuscitation (see page 45).

Prevention

• Healthy, fit dogs can drown due to fatigue if they are unable to get out of the water.
• If you have a swimming pool make sure the dog knows how and where to get out of it.

Ear Haematoma

Signs

• Ear haematoma is a circumscribed swelling of the ear flap containing blood. It is usually caused by the dog scratching and shaking its ear, or by a blow or bite from another dog that ruptures a blood vessel in the ear flap.

Action

• When the blood vessel in the ear flap first breaks, apply an icepack for 10 to 15 minutes to stop bleeding and reduce the swelling.
• If the swelling is small, apply pressure for 10 to 15 minutes with the thumb on one side of the ear flap and the index finger on the other.

• If the haematoma persists, take your dog to the veterinarian who will anaesthetise the dog and drain the haematoma. If the haematoma is not drained, the blood forms into a hard, fibrous swelling, distorting the shape of the ear, the same as a cauliflower ear seen in humans.

Eye Injuries

• Any injury to the eyeball or eyelids should be regarded as serious.
• Damage to the eyeball may lead to permanent blindness.
• Any break in an eyelid may lead to tear loss and a dry eye.
• Dogs with pop-eyes, such as a Pekingese, have a very shallow eye-socket in which the eye sits and, as such, the eye is more prone to injury and more prone to pop out of its socket.

Action

• Place a wad of cottonwool (absorbent cotton) soaked in water over the eye to keep eyelid(s) and/or eyeball moist.
• Seek veterinary attention immediately.

EYEBALL PROLAPSE
(EYE POPPED OUT OF THE SOCKET)

• Keep the eyeball moist with a cottonwool (absorbent cotton) ball soaked in water.
• Attempt to pull the eyelids over the protruding eyeball. If successful, apply even, firm pressure to push (do not force) the eyeball back into the socket.
• Seek veterinary attention immediately.

CHLORINE OR CEMENT BURNS TO THE EYE

Because the eye is moist, chlorine or cement will adhere to the eye, burning it and in some cases causing permanent damage or blindness.

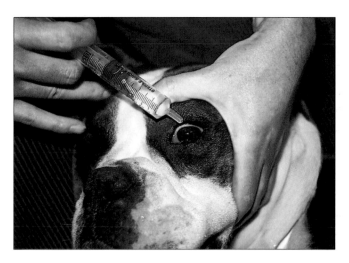

Wash chlorine or cement from the eye with a syringe filled with clean water.

• Wash the eye immediately and repeatedly, using such techniques as:

- A syringe filled with clean water.
- A very gentle stream of water from a hose.
- Wiping the eye gently until clean with a cottonwool (absorbent cotton) ball saturated in water, then dripping water onto the eye from a saturated cottonwool ball.

• Seek veterinary help quickly.

Foreign bodies such as a grass seed can cause permanent damage to the eye.

FOREIGN BODY IN THE EYE

Action

• Wash the eye with copious amounts of water.
• Gently open and close the eyelids to work the foreign body toward the corner of the eyelids or to make it visible.
• If visible, carefully attempt to remove the foreign body.
• If unable to remove, or if after removal the dog is very uncomfortable, seek veterinary assistance.
• Seek veterinary assistance if the dog's eye is tightly closed and you cannot identify the problem.

71

Fishhook Caught in Lip

Caution

• Do not push or pull the hook.

Action

If the dog is quiet and the barbed end of the hook is protruding through the lip

• With an assistant holding the dog's head very firmly to keep it still, cut through the hook with a pair of pliers or metal cutters at a point between the barb and the skin, or between the eye of the hook and the skin, whichever is the more convenient.
• The remainder of the hook can then be removed readily.

If the dog is agitated or the barbed end of the hook is embedded in the lip or mouth

• Seek veterinary assistance.

Fishing Line or Thread Disappearing into the Dog's Mouth

Caution

• Do not cut the line or thread. It may be attached to a fishhook or needle and could be of use to the veterinarian in locating and removing either of these objects.

Action

• Open the dog's mouth.
• If the fishing line or cotton disappears over the back of the tongue, gently pull the line or thread.
• If it will not budge, do not persist in pulling.
• Seek veterinary help.

Fit or Convulsion

- Lying on side.
- Unconscious.
- Paddling the legs.
- Champing the jaws.
- Frothing at the mouth.
- Twitching.

Do you know?

- The fit usually lasts for a minute or two, then the dog recovers.

Caution

- Do not try to take hold of the dog's tongue as you may be badly bitten by the champing jaws of the unconscious dog.

Action

- Observe the dog, but do not touch. Touching may prolong and aggravate the fit.
- Once recovered, the dog may seem a little disorientated. Make an appointment to see your veterinarian.
- If the dog continues fitting beyond five minutes, take the dog to your veterinarian immediately.
- If the dog is taking a series of fits, in between fits lift the dog gently into the car and go immediately to your veterinarian. (See pages 15 and 17.)
- If the dog is impossible to handle, call your veterinarian for help.

Do you know?

Dogs with pendulous ears covered with long hair are more susceptible to foreign bodies, the most common being grass seed.

Foreign Body in the Ear

Signs

- Shaking the head vigorously, frequently holding the head to one side and scratching the affected ear.

Action

- Check the ear flap inside and out.
- Get an assistant to hold the dog's head still.
- Use a torch to examine the ear canal and if discharge is

73

present, clean it out with a cotton bud (swab). If a foreign body is present, it usually comes away with the discharge.

• If the foreign body remains embedded, remove it with blunt-ended tweezers.

• Make sure you do not probe too deeply into the ear as you could do more harm than good.

• If you are unable to locate or remove a foreign body and the dog is distressed, see your veterinarian.

Fracture

Caution

• A fracture causes pain. A dog in pain may bite. So, if you are not sure, apply a muzzle (see page 41) before handling or moving a dog with a possible fracture.

• In giving First Aid your aim is to prevent the fracture and surrounding injured area from being worsened, especially during transit to the veterinary hospital.

• If the injured dog is in a danger zone, for example, a busy street, move the dog to a safe area for treatment.

Signs

• Swelling.
• Pain.
• Holding a limb off the ground.
• Limb(s) misshapen or dangling.
• Both hind legs are collapsed.
• Dog unable to move hind legs or all four limbs.

Action

For a leg fracture

• Apply a bandage using the Robert Jones technique: evenly wrap layers of cottonwool (absorbent cotton) around the leg, well above and below as well as over the fracture site. Very firmly wrap gauze bandage over the cottonwool, compressing it, and then cover the bandage and the nearby hair with adhesive bandage (see page 34).

• Lift and carry the dog to your car for transit to the veterinary hospital by hooking one arm under and around the neck and against the chest and the other arm under and around the abdomen.
• If the dog is too heavy to lift, place a blanket alongside and gently pull the dog onto the blanket by the scruff of the neck. With a person at each end taking hold of the corners, the blanket can be used as a stretcher to lift and carry the dog (see page 17).

> **Do you know?**
>
> The majority of fractures in the dog involve the limbs, pelvis, lower jaw or spine.

For a spine fracture

• If the dog cannot use the hind legs and there is no reaction when you pinch the toes, suspect a middle to lower spine fracture.
• If the dog cannot use the forelegs and hind legs, suspect a neck injury.
• *Very carefully* pull the dog by the scruff of the neck onto a blanket placed alongside (see page 17).
• Take the dog to your veterinarian.

Caution

• Transport the dog with minimal movement of its spine to prevent any further damage to the spinal cord.

For a pelvic fracture

• If the dog is unable to stand on the hind legs, there is a possible multiple fracture of the pelvis.
• If the dog is able to walk tentatively with the hind legs, there is a possible minor fracture.
• Lift and carry the dog as for a fractured leg (see above).
• Take the dog to your veterinarian.

For a jaw fracture

• Generally, fracture of the jaw does not require immobilisation.
• Take the dog to the veterinary hospital.

Types of fracture

Clean break A simple, clean-cut break

Greenstick Generally a bone fracture of young dogs where one side of bone is broken and the opposing side is intact.

Hairline A crack indicated by a fine line which may not be through the full thickness of the bone.

Impacted One fractured end of the bone forced into the other.

Multiple The bone is broken in two or more places.

Compound In a compound fracture, the fractured end of the bone protrudes through the skin. This is a serious fracture because of the danger of infection. Cover the wound with a gauze swab or clean linen cloth, for example, a handkerchief, then apply a bandage using the Robert Jones technique as described for a leg fracture (see page 34).

Frostbite

• Dogs exposed to temperatures below freezing point for lengthy periods are susceptible to frostbite.
• Dogs with short hair are more susceptible than others.
• The extremities, that is, the ears, toes, tail and scrotum, because of their poorer blood supply and greater exposure, are the sites most often affected.

Signs

• The skin is pale white in colour, very cold to the touch and loses its sensation.

Action

• If wet, dry the dog thoroughly.
• Wrap the dog in a thick, warm blanket.
• Warm the frostbitten area in a bath at approximately 40°C (104°F) for about 10 minutes.

• Apply a pad soaked in the same warm water (40°C or 104°F) to areas such as the tips of the ears.
• If the circulation returns, the skin will become red, swollen and look like a burn.
• Depending on the depth of the frostbite, if the circulation does not return, the skin will peel or a demarcation line will develop between the live and dead tissue.
• If the superficial skin layers only are peeling, apply a soothing antibiotic cream to soften the skin and control infection.
• If the tissues are pale, cold and insensitive after warming for 20 minutes, see your veterinarian.

Do you know?
• Prolonged heatstroke can lead to coma, brain damage or death.
• Dogs have no sweat glands and only regulate their body temperature by panting.

Heatstroke

Signs

• Panting.
• Mouth open, gasping for air.
• Distressed.
• Often unable to stand.
• Movement uncontrolled and agitated.
• Gums are deep red.

Action

• Cool the dog immediately by either wetting thoroughly with cold water, placing in front of a fan or in a cool, shady area with easy access to water as the dog improves.
• Seek veterinary help if the dog does not respond to treatment after 10 minutes.

Prevention

• Do not confine your dog in a poorly ventilated area in hot weather, for example, in a car with all the windows closed.
• Ensure your dog has access to cool water and a cool, shady area in very hot weather.

Hypothermia (Low Body Temperature)

A fullgrown healthy dog subjected to cold conditions normally does not suffer from hypothermia. However, keep in mind that the breed of dog and length of exposure to a certain temperature will have a bearing on whether or not the dog will suffer from hypothermia.

Hypothermia is most often observed in newborn puppies because they are unable to regulate their body temperature.

Signs

• Initially the puppy is restless, constantly crying and cold to the touch.
• Later the puppy becomes weak, stops crying and is uncoordinated. Sucking is weak or stops entirely.
• The dam (mother) rejects the pup.
• The puppy's temperature is 35°C (95°F) or less.

Action

• *Slow, gentle* heating, for example, with a hot water bottle, can lead to full recovery within 24 hours.

A puppy suffering hypothermia should be warmed gently and slowly to avoid shock.

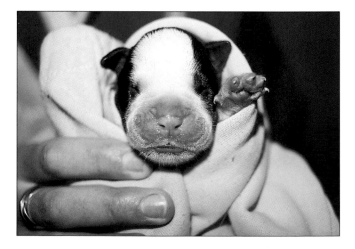

Caution

• Take care not to warm the puppy rapidly as this can lead to shock and death.

Hysteria

Some breeds, may become uncontrollably excited due to some external stimulation, for example, a thunderstorm.

Action

• If possible, remove the source of stimulation or the dog from the source.
• Encourage the dog to breathe with the nose just inside a plastic bag for a few minutes, thereby increasing the level of carbon dioxide in the blood. The bag is loosely held around the dog's nose so that air also can be inhaled.
• See your veterinarian who may tranquillise the dog and provide you with tranquillisers to give the dog prior to exposure to those stressful situations which produce hysteria. Tranquillisers should only be administered under strict veterinary direction.

Paralysis

• Dogs with short legs and long bodies, such as the Dachshund, Corgi and Pekingese, are prone to disc problems.
• These breeds and others, because of their conformation, can herniate (slip) a disc in the normal daily routine of running, jumping, twisting and turning in play.
• Severe traumas, such as caused by a motor vehicle accident, are common causes of spinal injury and paralysis.

Signs

- If the dog cannot use the hind limbs and there is no pulling away of the limbs when the toes are pinched, suspect a middle to lower spinal injury.
- If the dog cannot use the forelimbs and hind limbs and there is no response to pinching the toes, suspect a head or neck injury.

Action

- If the dog is lying quietly, gently pull the dog by the scruff of the neck onto a blanket placed alongside. With a person at each end holding the corners, the blanket can be used as a stretcher to lift and carry the dog (see page 17).

Caution

- Transport the dog to the veterinary hospital with minimal movement of the spine to prevent any further damage to the spinal cord.

Penis Protruding from Prepuce (Sheath)

Action

- Apply cold water or ice to the penis to reduce swelling.
- Carefully remove any long hairs around the opening of the sheath that may be causing an obstruction.
- Lubricate the penis and sheath opening with paraffin oil or another suitable lubricant.
- With your fingers, gently push the penis in as you pull the sheath out over the penis.
- If unsuccessful, seek the help of your veterinarian.

Poisoning

Signs

- The common signs are abdominal pain, salivating, vomit which may be tinged with blood, lethargy, diarrhea, burns about the mouth, reddening of the skin,

staggering, twitching, depression, convulsions and coma.
Only one or a few of these signs may be evident because
they vary according to the type of poison, the quantity
ingested and the length of time the dog has been
poisoned.

Action

• Telephone your veterinarian and describe the signs if
you are unsure of what has poisoned your dog. Some
countries have poison information centres which can
provide assistance.
• Initiate treatment *if you are sure* the dog has been
poisoned and you have identified the poison involved.

• See pages 82-87 for specific treatments of poisoning.
• See pages 57-60 for snake, tick and other bites.
• According to the poison involved, the treatment will
vary. It may be to:

1. Induce vomiting.
2. Wash the dog with soap and water then rinse if the
poisoning is external.
3. Give the dog copious amounts of water to drink.
4. Give special treatment such as medical oxygen,
resuscitation or antidote.

Using the poisons table

To use the poisons table on pages 82-87 you must be
sure that your dog has been poisoned and know what
poison is involved before giving treatment. If uncertain,
contact a veterinarian or poison information centre
immediately.

SPECIFIC TREATMENT FOR POISONS FOUND IN THE HOME AND GARDEN

Poison	Sources
Acids	Battery acids
Alcohol—Methylated spirits	An irresponsible person may offer a dog alcohol.
Anti-freeze (Ethylene glycol)	Used in car radiators; some dogs like the taste, will seek out and drink.
Arsenic (vermin, poisons, insecticides, herbicides)	Ingestion of grass sprayed or rodents poisoned with arsenical preparations; licking fur covered with insecticidal or herbicidal spray.
Aspirin (Acetylsalicylic acid)	Usually administered by owner without veterinary advice to alleviate pain or discomfort; a single large dose or a series of small doses can be poisonous.
Barbiturates, Sedatives, Anti-depressants	Sleeping tablets; valium.
Benzine hexachloride (Lindane, Dieldrin, Aldrin, Chlordane, Gammexane)	Insecticidal rinse for dogs in concentrated form.
Carbon monoxide	Car exhaust fumes; dog exposed to fumes if kept in garage.

Signs *(in order of onset or severity)*	Treatment
Burns on skin and mouth; vomiting may contain blood; shock.	If on skin, wash with warm water and soap, and rinse thoroughly and repeatedly with water. If ingested *do not* induce vomiting; give sodium bicarbonate (baking soda) in water and contact your veterinarian immediately.
Depression; wobbling; vomiting; collapse.	Give water; keep dog warm; contact your veterinarian.
Wobbling; vomiting; depression; convulsions; coma.	If sure that dog has ingested anti-freeze, induce vomiting (see page 88); take dog to your veterinarian who will inject ethyl alcohol to block effect of anti-freeze and administer further supportive treatment.
Salivating; thirsty; vomiting; fluid diarrhea with blood; abdominal pain; collapse; death.	Induce vomiting in early stages (see page 88); contact your veterinarian immediately who will administer antidote.
Signs vary according to period of time during which dosage administered; include poor appetite, depression, pale gums, vomiting, blood-tinged vomitus, staggering, falling over.	If recently administered, induce vomiting (see page 88); give sodium bicarbonate (baking soda) solution by mouth; contact your veterinarian.
Depression; wobbling; coma.	In early stages, induce vomiting (see page 88); contact your veterinarian.
Agitated; restless; twitching; convulsions; coma; death.	If no sign of convulsions, wash with soap and water and rinse thoroughly; contact your veterinarian.
Legs wobbly; breathing difficult; gums and mucous membrane around eyes (conjunctiva) bright pink.	Remove dog from poisonous environment to fresh air; if unconscious, give artificial respiration (see page 45); contact your veterinarian immediately who can administer oxygen directly to lungs with an endotracheal tube and give a respiratory stimulant.

SPECIFIC TREATMENT FOR POISONS FOUND IN THE HOME AND GARDEN

Poison	Sources
Chlorine	Concentrated powder or tablet used in swimming pools; chlorinated swimming pool water is not poisonous.
Kerosene	Heating fuel and cleaning fluid has a burning effect on dog's skin; dog licks affected area, thereby ingesting kerosene orally.
Lead	No longer used in paint manufacture, but some old houses still covered with lead paint; soil around lead mines polluted with lead; dog becomes poisoned by licking its coat contaminated with lead.
Metaldehyde	Snail and slug poison in powder or pellet form; dogs like the taste and actively seek it out.
Oil, grease	Dog lying under a motor vehicle or accidentally falling into a container.
Organo-phosphate carbomate	Snail and slug poison in pellet form; some dogs like the taste and will actively seek it out.
Paracetamol	Household pain reliever; may be administered to dog by owner.
Phenol (carbolic acid)	A potent disinfectant; poisonous to dogs by ingestion or absorption through skin; after skin contact, dog may ingest by licking the contaminated hair and skin.

Signs *(in order of onset or severity)*	Treatment
Weeping red eyes; salivating; red mouth; ulcerations of mouth and tongue; vomiting; diarrhea.	Rinse eyes and mouth with water; encourage dog to drink water; contact your veterinarian.
Red, inflamed skin; vomiting; diarrhea; possible convulsions; inflamed and ulcerated tongue.	Wash the dog's skin with soap and water; give the dog 20–30ml (2 tablespoons) of olive oil; contact your veterinarian.
Poor appetite; weight loss; vomiting; anaemic; diarrhea. Depending on degree of lead poisoning, dog may show signs of hyperexcitability, convulsions, depression, blindness, paralysis, coma.	Lead poisoning shows up over a period of time; consult your veterinarian who will confirm lead poisoning by a blood or urine test and will treat your dog with an antidote as well as for any presenting symptoms.
Tremor; salivation; diarrhea; wobbling; convulsions.	If dog observed at time of ingestion, induce vomiting (see page 88); contact your veterinarian immediately; recovery rate very good.
Covered in grease or oil; depressed.	Wash with warm water and soap; if unable to remove oil or grease, see your veterinarian.
Tremor; salivation; diarrhea; wobbling; convulsions.	If observed at time of ingestion, induce vomiting (see page 88); contact your veterinarian immediately; recovery rate very good.
May appear hours to days after ingestion. Include lethargy; gums may range from pale (anaemic) to yellow (jaundiced) to bluish; difficult breathing; swelling of lips and face.	Induce vomiting if recently ingested (see page 88); contact your veterinarian.
Dog smells of phenol; vomiting; diarrhea; severe abdominal pain; shock; collapse.	Remove phenol from hair and skin with soap and warm water; give 20–30ml (2 tblspns) of olive oil by mouth; contact your veterinarian.

SPECIFIC TREATMENT FOR POISONS FOUND IN THE HOME AND GARDEN

Poison	Sources
Strychnine	Rat poison, often used deliberately to poison animals with a bait.
Thallium	Rat, cockroach and ant poisons; dog can be poisoned by eating poisoned rat.
Turpentine (turps)	Paint solvent, wrongly used to remove paint from dog's hair or to dab on tick embedded in skin. Never use turps on dog's hair or skin as it can poison by absorption through skin.
Warfarin	The dog may eat the poison itself or eat a dead rat that has been poisoned with warfarin, which stops blood from clotting.

Signs *(in order of onset or severity)*	Treatment
Restless; twitching; general stiffness; convulsions with head and neck arched and limbs stretched out; convulsion can be set off by a touch or noise, become continuous, followed by death.	If dog has ingested strychnine, but shows no symptoms, induce vomiting immediately (see page 88). If showing symptoms, take to veterinarian immediately. In transit, do not touch dog or make a noise. If dog dies, strychnine can be confirmed by chemical analysis of stomach contents.
Vary according to amount ingested and period of time it is in dog's system. Redness of skin followed by a crust, peeling, and hair loss; starts on ears and lips, progresses to head, feet, limbs and body. Further symptoms are weight loss; vomiting; diarrhea; wobbling; convulsions.	Veterinarian can confirm by testing for thallium in urine. If dog has just swallowed thallium, induce vomiting (see page 88); see your veterinarian who will administer a drug to bind thallium and prevent its absorption through intestine.
Red, inflamed skin; dog vigorously licks skin affected by turps; vomiting; diarrhea; abdominal pain; restlessness; hyperexcitable; wobbly; coma.	Wash skin and hair with soap and water, rinse thoroughly; see your veterinarian.
Lethargy; pale gums and membrane around eye; weakness; laboured breathing; may be signs of haemorrhage in gum tissue; collapse; death. Signs may be slow to develop and vary according to time and amount ingested.	If recently ingested, induce vomiting (see page 88); treat for shock (see page 89); see your veterinarian who can administer an antidote; recovery rate very good.

1. Induce vomiting

Only induce vomiting for certain poisons (see pages 82-87), and if the dog is conscious and able to vomit. If the dog is unconscious or semiconscious when induced to vomit, it may inhale some of the vomit into the lungs causing death by asphyxiation or inhalation pneumonia. Give the dog Syrup of Ipecac (average adult dose is 2mls (⅓ teaspoon) per kg (2.2lb) of the dog's body weight). An alternative is 10 to 20mls (2 to 4 teaspoons) of a saltwater solution, concentration 3 teaspoons of salt to half a cup of warm water.

2. Wash the dog

Only wash the dog for certain poisons (see pages 82-87). If the dog's hair and skin are contaminated with a poisonous substance, wash the dog with warm water and soap, then rinse several times with plain water.

3. Give water to drink

Only give water to drink for certain poisons (see pages 82-87). If the dog has taken the poison internally via the mouth, give the dog copious amounts of water to drink. In the case of an acid, sodium bicarbonate solution is given if readily available. Where kerosene or phenol is ingested, 2 tablespoons of olive oil by mouth are recommended.

4. Special treatments

Consult your veterinarian about medical oxygen and antidotes. See page 45 for resuscitation.

Convulsions

• If the dog is convulsing intermittently, wait until the convulsions stop, then take the dog to your veterinarian together with a sample of the suspected poison, if available (see page 15 for handling).
• If the dog is convulsing continuously, try to prevent the

dog from self-injury by providing protective padding, for example, a folded blanket under the head. Avoid being bitten by handling the dog minimally, or by applying a muzzle (see page 41). Contact your veterinarian immediately for advice.

Prevention

• Make certain all toxic substances are kept out of reach.
• Use only clean containers for the dog's food and drinking bowls.
• In laying baits for vermin, slugs and snails or spraying the garden with herbicides and pesticides, make sure the dog has no access to the areas while the products are toxic.

Shock

• Shock is a term used to describe a state of collapse.
• Shock may range from mild to severe, and can bring about total collapse, coma and death.
• Shock usually results from some physical trauma often involving blood loss, poison, infection or dehydration.
• Shock is often evident in accident cases.

Signs

• Weakness, lying down.
• Rapid, weak pulse.
• Pale gums and conjunctiva.
• Rapid, shallow breathing.
• Cold to the touch.

Action

• Calm the dog.
• Keep the dog warm to maintain normal body temperature by wrapping the dog in a blanket, and/or by using a hot water bottle or heating pad.
• Control any bleeding (see page 61).
• In cases other than mild shock, take the dog to your veterinarian for immediate treatment.

Wounds

Wounds are classified as abrasions, contusions, incised wounds, lacerations and puncture wounds.

ABRASIONS
Signs

• The normal abrasion is painful to the touch, haemorrhages a little and more often than not is contaminated with debris.
• Caused by friction between the dog's body and a hard surface, such as a roadway. The hair and surface layer of skin, and sometimes the underlying tissues, are removed.

Action

Do you know?

Most wounds in dogs are contaminated and, as such, antibiotic treatment by your veterinarian should be considered.

• Clean the wound by spraying or by running water from a hose onto it. Water pressure should be sufficient to wash out debris but not so strong as to drive the debris into the damaged tissue. Alternatively, clean the wound initially with 3% hydrogen peroxide.
• When the wound is clean, pat it dry with clean gauze and dust or spray it with an antibiotic.
• Leave the abrasion open to the air to dry but if oozing freely cover with a gauze pad and bandage, and finally with an adhesive bandage until the oozing stops (see page 24).
• If the abrasion is left exposed to the air, use an Elizabethan collar (see page 32) so the dog cannot lick the wound.

Caution

• If the abrasion is deep, exposing bone, tendons, and so on, contact your veterinarian immediately.
• Vigorous and frequent licking of the wound will irritate it and slow down or prevent it from healing.

CONTUSIONS
Signs

• These wounds are characterised by bruising and swelling of the skin and underlying tissues. They are not necessarily associated with a break in the skin.
• Caused by a kick, fall or collision.

• If there is a break in the skin and you are aware of the contusion immediately after it appears, apply a cold compress. A swelling that has been present for some time and feels firm to hard is best dealt with by applying a hot foment (compress).

Action

Cold compress Hose the swollen area with a fair amount of water pressure or apply an ice pack for 30 minutes, repeating if necessary. The cold constricts the blood vessels and the pressure has a massaging effect.

Hot foment (compress) Pour hot water into a bucket containing 2 tablespoons of salt. The temperature of the water should be so hot that you can *just* put your hand into the water and keep it there. Soak a large wad of cottonwool (absorbent cotton) in the hot solution then hold it on the contused area until it cools off. Repeat for five minutes twice daily. The heat dilates the blood vessels helping to soften and disperse the swelling.

• If there is a break in the skin, see your veterinarian who will administer antibiotics.

INCISED WOUNDS

Signs

• Characteristics of these wounds are clean cut, fairly well opposed edges and minimum tissue damage.
• Caused by broken glass or similar sharp object.

Action

• If bleeding, apply pressure directly to the wound with a clean gauze pad or similar item until the bleeding stops.
• Clean the wound only if necessary.
• Gently but firmly pinch the opposing edges of the wound together.
• Apply thin strips of adhesive bandage in a crisscross formation about 1cm (0.5in) apart directly across the wound.
• Place a gauze pad over the wound. Secure with a gauze bandage held in place by an adhesive bandage. This will help to immobilise the edges of the wound (see page 24).
• Confine the dog.

• Leave the bandage in place for 48 hours, then check the wound.
• If the wound is clean, dry and showing no sign of inflammation, rebandage and change every 48 hours.

Caution

• If the wound is extensive (long and/or deep), contact your veterinarian to have it stitched.
• Such a wound should be stitched within eight hours.

LACERATIONS
Signs

• The wound edges are often irregular, jagged and gaping. Sometimes whole sections of the skin and underlying tissues are torn away.
• Lacerations are usually not painful and haemorrhage is variable.
• Caused by barbed wire, sharp edge of a tin, and so on.

Action

• Thoroughly clean the wound by hosing it or by applying 3% hydrogen peroxide.
• Remove any hair, dead tissue or foreign bodies from the wound.
• Apply antibiotic powder.
• Cover the wound with a gauze pad then a gauze bandage, both held firmly in place by an adhesive bandage (see page 24).
• See your veterinarian as the laceration may need to be stitched.
• If unable to be stitched, leave the bandage in place for two days.
• When the bandage is removed, hose the wound to clean away any discharge, debris or dead tissue and dress as before.
• Continue the bandaging until fleshy tissue has filled in the cavity to skin level. Then leave the bandage off, allowing the air and sunshine to dry the surface of the wound.
• If the dog licks the wound excessively, apply an

Elizabethan collar (see page 32).
• Restrict exercise until the skin has completely covered the wound.

• Carefully clip the hair away from the hole.
• Carefully check the wound to see that no foreign body remains embedded.
• Clean the area with 3% hydrogen peroxide and dab the wound with tincture of iodine.
• Do not allow a seal to form over the wound. Keep the wound open as long as possible while drainage is taking place.
• If the puncture appears to penetrate through the skin into the underlying tissues, take your dog to your veterinarian who will administer antibiotics and provide drainage if necessary.

PUNCTURE WOUNDS
Action

Do you know?

• Puncture wounds are often painful and may or may not be accompanied by haemorrhage.
• They can be caused by penetration of the skin by a splinter, piece of wire or nail, or eye (canine) tooth penetration in a fight.

INDEX